AWAKENING

THE GENIUS WITHIN

THE CULMINATION IN CELLULAR NUTRITION

by Roland Thomas, BSc, ND

foreword by Doctor Michael Kiriac, PhD, ND

DEDICATION

This book is dedicated to those who have suffered from the radiation ills of Chernobyl, and to all who suffer and struggle with illness. May you find health, happiness and above all, peace.

DISCLAIMER

This booklet is intended for educational and informational purposes only. The authors do not suggest that readers self-diagnose and / or self-medicate without the sound judgment and seasoned counsel of a well-informed healthcare provider. We strongly urge the reader to consult an appropriately educated practitioner before making any changes to health maintenance or therapeutic regimens.

Telephone : +1 303 683 8113
Web site: www.awakeningthegeniuswithin.com
Email: info@awakeningthegeniuswithin.com

ISBN: 1-890252-25-5 - Fifth Edition, January 2009 – formerly published under the title "The Magic of Bio-Algae Concentrates: The Life of Michael Kiriac"

Published by:
Quantum Leap Wellness Publishing

Designed and edited by:
Rodika Kiriac and Cornel Chiriac

CONTENTS

ACKNOWLEDGEMENTS

During the development of Bio-Algae Concentrates (BAC) my life has been dedicated to furthering the science and use of these God-given micro-algae nutrients for the health and survival of mankind. I would like to thank former-President Mikhail Gorbachev for his tenacious moral and financial support during the development of the concentrates amidst many political critics in the USSR.

I would like to thank my extraordinary teachers in Ukraine and Moldova and my close associates V. Rudic, I. Scutaru, and O. Sandu, as well as the many scientific partners who participated in the research and application throughout the development years. I also thank the numerous clients and health professionals for their testimonials and their trust in Cellular Nutrition. My special appreciation goes to Roland Thomas for his encouragement and support in the publication of this booklet. I especially acknowledge my adorable wife Liudmila for her support, her love, and her constant collaboration, and my daughters Rodika and Stefana, for their love and support.

Michael Kiriac, PhD, ND

I want to first acknowledge Dr. Michael Kiriac for the breakthrough development of the most advanced nutraceutical superfood available on earth at this time. For more than 20 years Michael Kiriac developed theories, performed the research, and made discoveries to produce the final product available today for humanity's benefits. I want the reader to know of Dr. Kiriac's heroic contributions to the cause of children and adults sick from the radiation of the Chernobyl disaster. I have known about the benefits of micro algae for many years, but Dr. Kiriac's influence has taken my appreciation for Bio-Algae Concentrates' place in human health to a new level of understanding. Dr. Kiriac has made groundbreaking contributions to the wellness of humanity.

I want to thank my many friends and clients for sharing their experiences with me. It is their well-being and encouragement that makes my journey rewarding.

Finally, I thank my wife and best friend Linda and my daughters Maryse and Myriam for their unwavering support and understanding, making each of my days worth living for.

Roland Thomas, BSc, ND

FOREWORD

All my life I have researched and applied nutrition as a solution to health and prevention of diseases. Thirty years ago I became convinced that nutrition was the foundation of health, which encourages the metabolic system to operate optimally.

I learned that ensuring proper cellular nutrition is more complex than just eating well and avoiding excess in our diet. It is more than adding a few vitamins, healthy foods, juices, and nutritional supplements. This will not make much of a difference when our body is already compromised by daily toxin attacks from pollutants in the air, water, and foods.

Some of the nutrients that we consume are absorbed into our body through the villi of the small intestine (see side notes). Most people assume that our bodies absorb all nutrients efficiently and completely. Unfortunately, nutrient absorption is greatly diminished or impaired by the state of our health, by stress, and by what we consume. This is because we are cellular beings – made up of trillions of specialized cells. Each cell is powered by a series of chemical reactions, such as the Krebs cycle, which supply the energy that every cell needs to carry out its activities. This process requires nutrients, including carbohydrates, amino acids, vitamins, minerals, and trace elements. Therefore, proper cellular nutrition ensures that the trillions of cells in our bodies are energized as best as possible, allowing the cells to grow, repair, and perform their functions efficiently. As a result we feel and look better, prevent and fight diseases, and control our weight.

THE VILLI OF THE SMALL INTESTINE

The small intestine has features designed to maximize food absorption. Most obvious is its length – about 22 feet long. It is coiled upon itself and packed neatly into the abdominal cavity. Its inside surface, about 1½ inches in diameter, is folded and ridged to further increase the surface and absorption area.

A closer look reveals that these folds and ridges are covered with millions of tiny finger-like projections called villi. Under a microscope, the surface of the cells lining the villi display the individual absorptive cells bristling with even smaller finger-like projections called the microvilli. If the small intestine were a simple featureless tube it would have had an inside surface area of several square yards, however, the microvilli increase the absorption surface to hundreds of square yards.

The principles of proper cellular nutrition are absorption and regeneration, which lead to all-important cleansing and critical hypothalamic function.

Absorption. The chemical breakdown of foods begins in the mouth with the actions of enzymes from the saliva. It continues along the digestive tract to the small intestine, where most digestion and absorption of nutrient molecules take place. Food particles drift around the villi of the intestinal microvilli, where various enzymes digest them until they are small enough to pass through the villi and into the bloodstream.

However, with most people, much of the nutrients from their foods never get into the bloodstream because the villi are often destroyed by salt, sugar, fat, tobacco, alcohol, chemicals, medicine, pollution, and stress. The energetically-impaired villi break off and become ineffective.

Regeneration. The body is constantly regenerating at the cellular level. For example, the villi are replaced every three days when there are enough nutrients absorbed to rebuild the villi. Since absorption is generally compromised in most people, there is a degenerative downward spiral that only gets worse because each new generation of villi are created more slowly. The poor absorption also compromises the continuous generation of new cells in the heart, lungs, muscles, brain, bones, and the rest of the body, creating cells of lesser vitality.

Cleansing. Compounding the problem, our Western lifestyles put tremendous toxic strain on our vital organs and glands. The stomach is perpetually stuffed with denatured foods of incompatible combinations. The liver is strained and even swollen while breaking down massive intakes of animal protein and fat as well as the associated drugs and poisons in the animal products. The pancreas balloons to abnormal size due to the over-demand for digestive enzymes to process enzyme-deficient foods. The villi and microvilli may break off and clog up the digestive tract, and the colon becomes lined with layers of glue-like undigested foods that poison the bloodstream.

Because of poor nutrition, incomplete absorption, and slow cellular regeneration, the blood and other tissues accumulate toxins and gradually lose their vitality. If we do not purge ourselves of these toxins regularly, toxicity becomes worse until the body either purges itself spontaneously – diarrhea, acne, pimples, boils, liver spots, foul perspiration, body odor, bad breath, and so forth – or it simply gives up the battle and succumbs to degenerative conditions.

Hypothalamus. The main metabolic body-balancing control system in the body is the hypothalamus, located at the base of the brain and atop of the spinal column. It connects to the organs and glands in a synergistic two-way communication. Via the bloodstream, it receives its own very important nutrients, as well as status and requests from all the cells in the rest of the body. When the hypothalamus itself is poorly fed, it does its own job less effectively, contributing to the downward spiral, becoming less and less able to regulate the glands that control all metabolisms and to respond to the requests by the cells to perform the myriad of their other functions.

Mother Nature will ultimately sentence anyone who consistently breaks the laws of nature to chronic disease and premature death. The number of people in their 40s, 50s and 60s with serious health problems that lead to heart attacks, cancers, and strokes is staggering, augmenting, and unnecessary.

When I came to Canada, I realized that in my homeland, the former USSR, we had a better quality of nutrition since we lived closer to the land – fresher, more natural foods, and less pollution. Only in the ravages of the Chernobyl nuclear disaster did I see the level of the degenerative diseases – cancer, diabetes, osteoarthritis, allergies, and immune system disorders – the diseases that I found in North America. Why is that? Poor nutrition is the major cause.

In this booklet you will learn that Bio-Algae Concentrates (BAC) regroup thousands of naturally occurring, balanced, and synergistic nutrients to overcome the inefficiencies and blockages in the digestive system. BAC increases nutrient absorption, enhances regeneration of all cells, including those of the villi and the microvilli in the small intestine, reduces the load on the cleansing organs of the body, and awakens the hypothalamus. This in turn triggers cellular awakening and metabolic healing in the trillions of cells in your body. The downward spiral towards disease is reversed into an upward spiral back to health and vitality, boosting your immune and nervous systems and other vital organs.

The end result – you will feel the difference!

Michael Kiriac, Montreal, December 2002

BRINGING LIGHT TO THE SHADOW OF DEATH

It was 1949. Michael Kiriac's mother, Stefana, was horribly worried for the whole family. Stefana's father had just died young of pancreatic cancer. Eleven years earlier, the same cancer had claimed the life of her son Simion at age twelve. This kind of genetic weakness often decimated families in the region. Her fears for her family, born and unborn, materialized in a series of tragic deaths from pancreatic cancer. Michael Kiriac was destined to finally stop the tragedies for his family and thousands of other families – but it took 40 years. His magnificent story follows.

Michael was born in 1952 in Kishinev, Moldova, then part of the Union of Soviet Socialist Republics (USSR), as the youngest of ten children in a single-story, three-bedroom house. His father, Ignat, worked as a laborer on the local farms. Michael loved his father, who was healthy, strong and worked hard all his life.

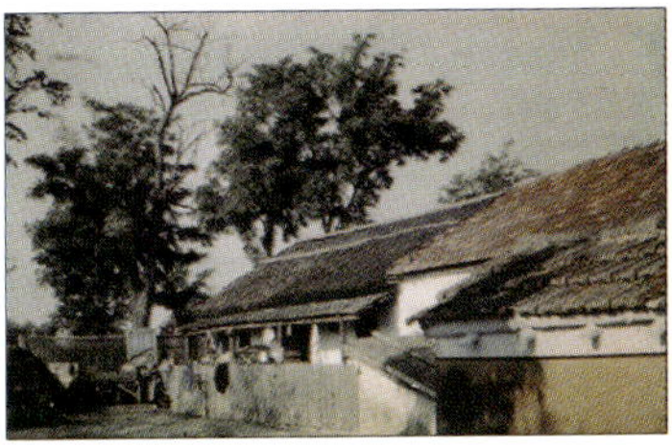

MICHAEL KIRIAC'S CHILDHOOD HOME

A poor but simple country lifestyle provided the opportunity to live close to the land, eat fresh home-grown foods, and fast at times, according to the local orthodox religious traditions. His many older siblings challenged and tutored him from a young age, accelerating his early learning and fueling his innate curiosity of nature's fascinating ways.

From an early age Michael began to help family members, neighbors, and friends with headaches, back problems, and other maladies. He learned to employ diverse local herbs, oils, recipes, herbal blends known as poultices, as well as Bioenergetics – a hands-on energy modality. Michael was already demonstrating a remarkable understanding of what bodies need for health.

In the continuing family tragedy, Ignat Kiriac was diagnosed with pancreatic cancer in August of 1964 and died a few months later. Nothing could be done – the disease was sudden and death was rapid. It shook everyone in the family.

The family had been dependent on father's salary, even though the USSR's system supported their housing. Shock and doom swept the whole family, leaving young Michael astounded that all the discoveries and progress of science were powerless to stop the tragedy. Filled with burning questions about cancer, life and death, and the shortcomings of medical science, he resolved to devote his life to the search for answers.

THE ROAD TO DISCOVERY

Four years later, Michael, with a high school diploma in hand, was eager to absorb everything the Moldova Academy of Sciences could teach him about disease and health.

DISCOVERING NUTRITION AS THE WAY TO HEALTH

After three years of intensive study in Human Anatomy, Physiology, and Biology, Michael began to realize that we are cellular beings, nourished by other cells of nature, and that Nutrition has the potential to surpass the "break and fix" approach to medicine by preventing degeneration and empowering cells to thrive as nature intended them to do.

During that time period Soviet policy demanded research to be done at many universities to end the pandemic of cancers running rampant throughout Eastern Europe and Western USSR in the 1970's. The Moldova Academy of Sciences agreed with Michael's professors that his desire to focus on organic nutrition was worthy and sponsored research at his university, beginning a long and fruitful association that would give him superior research opportunities.

He focused his research on identifying foods that would far exceed the modest results that raw, organic and green natural foods had already been shown to provide. Michael knew then that he could make a difference in people's lives and he decided to dedicate his life to health via natural nutrition. To that end, he took a degree in Cellular Nutrition in 1973.

SUPER NUTRITION IN ALGAE

After graduation, the Moldova Academy of Sciences put Kiriac to work on several research projects in the region, and also encouraged him to pursue his own research while continuing his studies.

As part of his research, he attended lectures on then current Japanese scientific research and studied papers describing positive results with Chlorella. It was then that he decided to begin his research efforts with this micro-alga. See the side note "What are micro-algae?".

Today algae are being used by millions of humans and animals around the world. They are known to boost health, effectively avoiding the need for antibiotics to combat infections.

During his early research, hundreds of trials and tests using the Chlorella alga showed good results in reduction of

WHAT ARE MICRO-ALGAE?

Everything humans need to live in good health already exists on Earth. One of the most healthful foods is spread in a fine film over most of the surface of the earth, invisible to the naked eye. However, modern intelligent humans have lost sight of its value. Ancient humans, Aztecs, Mayans, tribal Africans, the largest mammals (whales) and other intuitively intelligent animals have long been aware of this natural life-giving food source. The plant cells in this film are called micro-algae.

These little organisms are miniature factories, turning out amazing amounts of nutrients such as vitamins, minerals, protein, and enzymes. Some species contain more nutrition per ounce than anything you can eat, including bee pollen, which is the most nutritionally dense land-based food.

There are over 25,000 species of algae on earth

cancers in cattle, sheep, and goats, but not in chickens, rabbits, pigs, or horses. This led to an important realization that the latter species could not digest Chlorella properly due to its cell membrane being made of cellulose, which requires the enzyme cellulase for proper digestion.

After two years of research with the Chlorella alga, he began investigating hundreds of other algae with strong emphasis placed on several different strains of the Spirulina algae, which at the time had shown promising results.

Directed research techniques were applied allowing him to accomplish hundreds of precise tests with conclusive results. For example, at times he and his researchers worked with more than 250 test groups of 30 - 40 animals per group.

SEARCHING FOR THE BEST ALGAE

From 1973 to 1977, during the intensive search for the best algae, more than one thousand different species of micro-algae were selected from all over the world and tested for their individual benefits as well as for their complimentary and synergistic combination potential. For example, over 65 strains of Spirulina alone were involved in experimentation.

and thousands of micro-algae, and more are discovered each year. Many contain a higher concentration of chlorophyll than any other known plant, and have a very complex RNA and DNA. Some micro-algae are a complete protein food, containing large amounts of beta-carotene (provitamin A), all the B vitamins, vitamin C and E, and many minerals in high enough amounts to be considered perfect food. Most importantly, the essential amino acid profile of algae is virtually identical to that required by the human body.

Certain micro-algae are effective in eliminating heavy metals, such as lead, mercury, copper, and cadmium. The protein yield is greater than soybeans, corn, and beef. Some algae contain GLA, a very important essential fatty acid and a precursor to the body's master hormones. Research has shown that Spirulina algae alone could double the complete protein available to humanity on a fraction of the world's land. Acre for acre, Spirulina yields 20 times more protein than soybeans and 400 times more protein than beef. Its makeup is 71% protein, 17% carbohydrates, and 7% fats.

Several types of micro-algae stimulate the immune system, improve digestion, detoxify the body, enhance growth and tissue repair, accelerate healing, protect against radiation, help prevent degenerative disease, and promote longer life. They may strengthen the liver, the body's major detoxifying organ. Many have a beneficial effect on arthritis and hypertension. One example of a most important benefit comes from a combination of molecules that biochemists call the Controlled Growth Factor, a unique composition that provides a noticeable increase in sustained energy and immune health when eaten regularly.

Various blue, green, and red algae were also used, including the carotenoid-rich Dunaliella and Astaxanthin-rich Haematococcus, selected for their superior antioxidant powers. Astaxanthin alone may carry up to 1,000 times the antioxidant power found in Vitamin E and up to 40 times more than that found in carrots.

Dr. Kiriac and his team rapidly achieved significant results using various concentrations of base algae, such as Spirulina and Dunaliella.

As was customary in the former USSR, research always began with laboratory mice and rats before proceeding to larger species like poultry, ducks, rabbits, pigs, and cattle. When research demonstrated to be safe, it proceeded to humans.

With mice and rats responses were rapid due to their natural extraordinary metabolic strength. It proved more difficult with the larger animals. The results, though promising, were not efficient or rapid enough to stir up the team. They knew that a breakthrough blend was necessary to help the larger animals.

ANOTHER TRAGEDY TURNS FOCUS TO HUMAN SOLUTIONS

Tragedy again struck the Kiriac family in 1977. Michael's first-born, Julian, fell ill and died at four months. Not until then was it discovered he had a systemic endocrine cancer. His devastated family was resigned that it was the unfortunate genetic disposition to the glandular cancer his parents and many siblings suffered.

But not Michael; he was convinced that he could make a difference with nature's complete nutrition. From then on, his research focus turned to human solutions as much as possible. He knew that dramatically improving the health of the cells in humans would not only affect their health but also that of the DNA within the cells. Further, genetic transmission from cell to cell is influenced by the central nervous system. Excellent nutrition creates better memory in the nervous system and therefore in the DNA.

Michael believed that cellular and genetic health, as well as a stronger immune system, could be passed on to his future children through their mother, Liudmila. He was determined more than ever to find the correct combination of micro-algae to not only remedy cancers and other diseases and conditions, but to prevent fatal illnesses in his family. His wife was among the first to receive the new micro-algae formula as it was developed, leading to her excellent health and their yet-to-be born daughters.

Mr. Kiriac had narrowed down his research to two strains of Spirulina (for their high content of naturally-occurring proteins, vitamins, minerals and enzymes), Dunaliella (for its exceptional vitamin C and mixed antioxidant content) and Astaxanthin (for its superior antioxidant power). However, when the algae were used singly, the cancers were not eradicated quickly enough or with enough consistency. New significant steps were yet to be made when, for example, it was concluded that any single base alga by itself lacked either sufficient vitamin C or zinc, or some other co-factor for maximum assimilation of its nutrients, minerals, enzymes, or antioxidants to effectively combat cancer and other degenerative conditions.

AMAZING PRODUCTION WITH BIOREACTORS

In 1978, the first of many extraordinary incidents occurred which led to a significant advancement in the algae research and their growth technologies. One night, the lights in the hydroponic basin – known as the bioreactor, were left on by mistake, exposing the algae culture to light for a longer period of time. The next morning, the algae color had changed from its usual dark green to a new reddish tint – the color of beta-carotene. The algae had increased in beta-carotene content because of the overexposure. This simple discovery led to many more experiments applying various changes to the base environment, such as light exposure, tem-

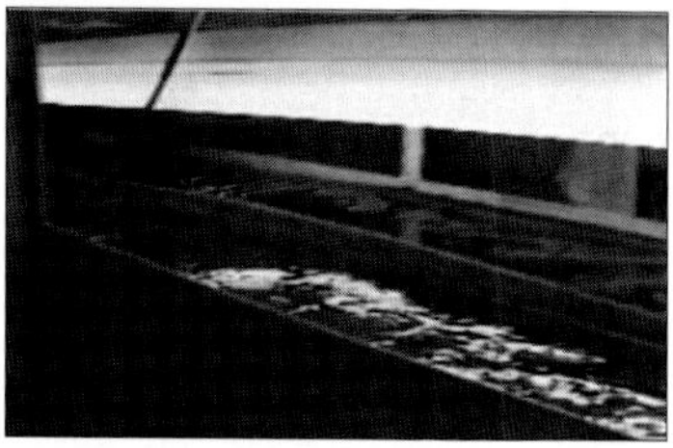

RESEARCH BIOREACTOR
Creating technology to grow algae efficiently in a controlled environment

perature, turbulence, nutrients, and duration of exposures.

These experiments resulted in the controlled increase or decrease of various combinations of nutrients in the algae: alpha and beta-carotene, sodium, zinc, selenium and several beneficial vitamins and minerals.

EUREKA! BIO-ALGAE CONCENTRATES – SUPERNUTRITION

With the culmination of several years of research, the resulting micro-nutrient algae concentrates were coined Bio-Algae Concentrates (BAC). Compared to the earlier, simpler algae blends, the BAC nutraceutical powers were far superior. See side note "How are BAC Compared to Algae?"

It was rewarding working with BAC combinations when applied to mice, rats, ducks, chickens, and rabbits because of their rapid healing effects on the animals. Several test breeds reproduced multiple times within one year, enabling researchers to quickly observe the effect on the next generations.

During this exciting discovery period, Mr. Kiriac realized his dream: the proper mix and dose of BAC would help the prevention and recovery from many diseases for humans as well as for animals. Thousands more tests, trials, and applications were carried out with cancer-ill mice, rats, chickens, rabbits, and pigs, as well as with cattle, which in Europe were affected by leukemia.

His ultimate realization was "that what was really at work was the self-healing power of the body in combination with super nutrients". Given the enormous offering of nutrients that are naturally occurring in BAC's balanced and synergistic blend, the body's innate capacity is triggered to take what it needs to nourish and self-repair. BAC targets the brain glands via super nutrition, in particular the hypothalamus, pituitary, and pineal, because only they and the central nervous system they control are able to powerfully awaken a sluggish immune system. This discovery and research results

HOW ARE BAC COMPARED TO ALGAE?

BAC are a breed apart from plain algae because of the completeness, the balance, and the synergies obtained from its selected algae when blended in precise proportions. Each alga in the blend is selected for its base nutritional value, and, with advanced hydroponics, nurtured to its peak nutritional potential:

- Spirulina Pacifica and Platensis have the broadest number of proteins, vitamins, minerals, EFA, trace elements, and enzymes naturally occurring on Earth.
- Astaxanthin, derived from Haematoccocus Pluvialis, is believed to be the alga that can accumulate the highest levels of antioxidants in nature. Many studies show that it is the most powerful natural antioxidant on Earth.
- Dunaliella is a green or yellow mono-cellular alga that contains the highest known concentration of beta-carotene: minimally 10% of the base alga weight. Dunaliella has been used in anti-cancer research and has many promising results in reduction of tumors and cancer cells. It is also very high in vitamin C, which complements Spirulina's low content. Data suggests there is critical synergy between Spirulina and vitamin C.

The final BAC product contains over 5,000 known nutrient constituents and is 100% natural – not artificial. BAC's high protein content averages 50%, with 98-99% net utilization. BAC contains many phytonutrients, nature's special forces such as lycopene, phycocyanin, chlorophyll, polysaccharides, sulfolipids, and others; Essential Fatty Acids (EFA) – Omega 3, 6 and 9 – and linoleic acid (GLA); thousands of active natural enzymes; powerful antioxidants such as Astaxanthin, which has hundreds of times the antioxidant activity of vitamin E and 40 times that of carrots; the vitamins A, B-complex, B12, C, E, D; all essential amino acids; all known minerals and trace elements like calcium (with 95-98% net were published within the Academy of Science. By then, Mr. Kiriac was driving his research towards solutions for pancreatic cancer in several animal populations with the intent to resolve this disease for the remaining members of his family. His personal motivation to find cures for pancreatic cancer led to extensive research and the development of many BAC formulations throughout these productive years.

assimilation), zinc, sodium, iron, phosphorus, and potassium, etc.

BAC are a perfect example of the saying "the whole is larger than the sum of its parts." BAC are exponentially more nutritionally efficient than plain alga such as Spirulina or Chlorella, and because of that, have significantly more nourishing, rejuvenating, and healing effects on the body and brain.

MOTHER'S CANCER BRINGS INSPIRATION

In 1984, while Mr. Kiriac was nearing confirmation of the optimum combinations of algae and of the technologies of the base solutions in his research, his mother was diagnosed with pancreatic cancer. She attempted to combat the cancer with his latest concepts and knowledge – using raw foods, wheat grass juice, and Spirulina – but not the algae formula, since it was not perfected for humans at that time. She tragically succumbed to cancer at the age of 80. It had seemed so possible that his research and efforts could have saved her. This further demonstrated the strong genetic tendency to pancreatic cancer in the family and brought gloom to the remaining family members.

After his mother's death, Michael turned his pain and heartache into even more determined action and inspiration. He knew he was close to a breakthrough that could save the rest of his family. He worked day and night with hundreds of animal test groups.

Finally, after this extremely hard work, many years and thousands of clinical tests, his team had narrowed their focus exclusively on the red Haematococcus algae for its potent Astaxanthin, on the orange Dunaliella for its mix carotenoids, and on the two of the best Spirulina for their broad and complementary nutrient spectrum. Precise enhancements and combinations of these four prime algae provided the long-awaited blends with superior balance and synergy.

From this point forward, success with larger animal species was rapid as BAC delivered much more potent and absorbable nutrition immediately to cells. The health of both large and small animal populations was consistently stabilized in four to six weeks, and for many, remission would occur rapidly after due to the innate power that fully nourished and empowered cells to cleanse themselves and split into healthier child cells. During those years, parallel experiments and practical applications with humans were ongoing with the researchers themselves and the local medical clinics. Michael became known as a brilliant young scientist and contributor to the future of mankind. His discoveries had spread in scientific circles as far as Moscow, including the Academy of Science and the Ministry of Nutrition.

VALIDATED SUPER NUTRITION EXPANDS TO MILLIONS OF TEST ANIMALS

In 1985, after completing ten years of intense research focusing on the science of algae applied to cancers and other diseases with the Academy of Science of Moldova, Kiriac was enthusiastically invited to join the Ministry of Agriculture of Moldova as chief of the Nutrition Sciences department. They asked him to accelerate his research for application to the agriculture industry, specifically livestock.

A large poultry farm in Moldova was selected to be the research center. He spent the next eleven years working with this facility, even while on other assignments and managing other projects. He continues to collaborate with the facility up to this day.

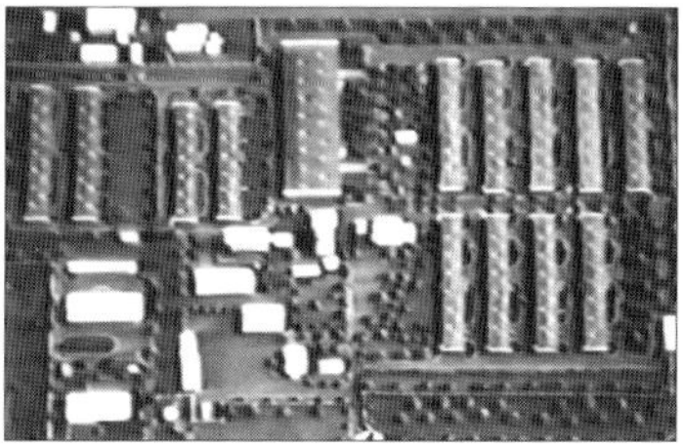

RESEARCH CENTER
Facilities for 600 workers, 200 researchers, 1.5 million egg-laying chickens in 20 buildings

Housing and research facilities were established for 600 workers and 200 researchers. The research center hosted up to 1½ million egg-laying chickens in several buildings surrounding the main research facility, each holding 75,000 chickens.

Mr. Kiriac later remarked that this facility alone raised more chickens than half the population of chickens found in the entire province of Quebec, Canada. This was unheard of elsewhere because of the danger of epidemic diseases wiping out all the chickens at once. But this did not worry Mr. Kiriac since BAC was being applied to the chicken feed, resulting in consistently disease-free chickens.

The research center's mandate was to:

- House the largest, most technologically-advanced algae bioreactor facility on Earth
- Eradicate and prevent diseases on the farm, including cancers such as the Marek disease
- Increase animal productivity
- Be as biologically organic as possible
- Derive profits through selling animal products to other countries

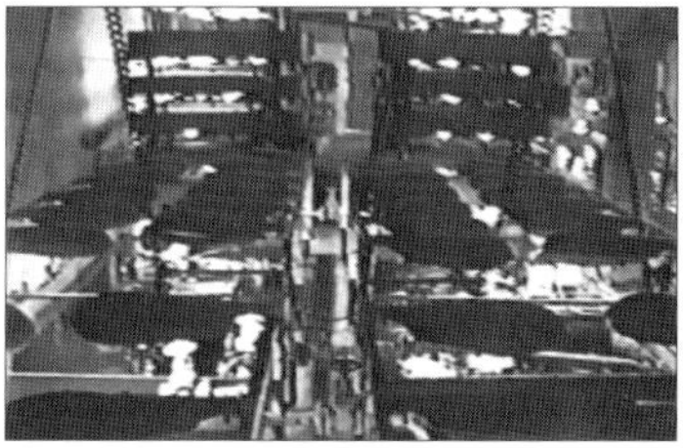

BIOREACTORS
Several 5 sq m surfaces – each providing as much as 25 acres of open farm land and delivering more nutrients in a perfectly controlled environment

Over the years, the project was able to achieve astounding animal health. For example, the poultry achieved 100% healing and eradication of the Marek disease, saving 100% of the diseased animals. About 50% of the newly-healed animals where returned to the production cycle to lay eggs again. All this was achieved with the use of organic grains and BAC, without the use of antibiotics, growth hormones, or other artificial means. By using BAC, farms gained superior productivity in production farming of poultry for meat and eggs in Moldova, Ukraine, and Russia, as demonstrated by:

- 20% overall productivity increase
- Increase in viability of the chickens by 4.45%
- Increased chicken average weight by 21.26%
- Diminished feed by 14%
- Increased strength of the eggshell
- Rise of 5.8% in egg fertilization
- Rise of 3.8% in egg laying
- Decreased mortality rate of chicks to 1.35% from an average of 10%
- Larger eggs with stronger shells
- 24 versus 17 months of laying egg period
- 14 more eggs per month per chicken
- Better tasting meat and eggs

In addition, extensive use of BAC by the farm workers contributed to better health, less absenteeism, and higher productivity.

Reaching its organic goals, everything produced from the chickens was used or re-used, such as eggs, meat, egg powder, and chicken droppings as organic fertilizer.

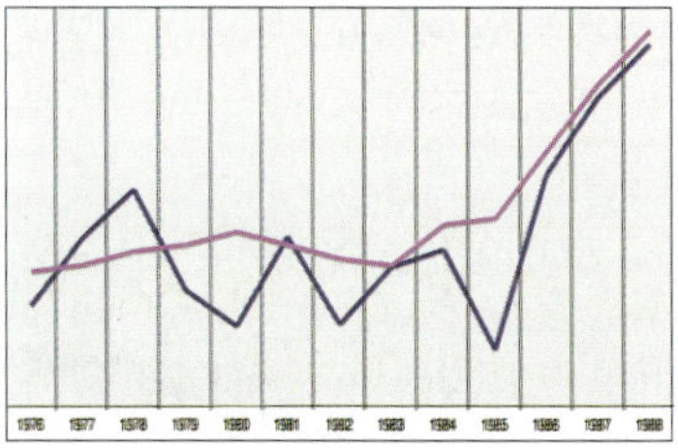

POULTRY PRODUCTIVITY 1976 - 1988
After devastation by Marek desease to a nine-year low in 1985, Mr. Kiriac's new methods and BAC dramatically raised productivity

The farm also became economically viable. Poultry-derived products – egg powder, chicken meat, eggs, and poultry droppings – were sold in several countries: Germany, Holland, Bulgaria, Austria, and Vietnam.

In two years, it was observed and confirmed that when applying BAC to the first generation of poultry, the subsequent generation became healthier and the next generation even healthier, stronger and more resistant to diseases. The second and subsequent generations did not suffer from cancers.

The farm allowed for extensive directed technology research because of the large population of chickens available as test groups. Mr. Kiriac was able to use part or all of the huge populations in each building to further prove the value of BAC, which constituted a major leap in global research. Most clinical research with animals is normally limited to 40 - 100 test animals, but he was able to compare BAC's results in large populations of 28,000 – 83,000 chickens to another large test group of similar size. Each test group was verified for diverse signs of health, such as longevity, birth rates, food taste, animal size, and number of eggs.

The optimum dosage was introduced in the industry immediately, resulting in a productivity increase. At that time, this project had become a major priority for the USSR. Budgets were approved for continued research in the production technologies and the final BAC formulations. This support allowed for the significant advances and precise formulation of the recipes.

This success was highly rewarding and motivating for Mr. Kiriac, who by then wanted to convert the world to this kind of organic health. To this day, he remembers the delicious taste of the chicken meat and of the eggs, even when eaten raw. The success and the health recovery were so unparalleled, that he was eager to develop BAC for humans to help with the cancer crisis and to protect his family.

The benefits continued unabated. Biological farming with BAC as feed supplement led to planning for the development of the largest BAC production centers in Europe: Moldova, Voronezh and Moscow in Russia, Omsk and Kamchatka in Siberia. The large, hydroponic bioreactor allowed for year-round production, independent of the weather and the sun, capable of producing far greater volume of higher-grade algae due to the easy control of the base culture used. This greatly reduced the space needed for algae production. One liter of harvested algae paste delivered thousands more nutrients than that found in 25 acres of Alfalfa. Alfalfa was used extensively for poultry feed because of its many nutrients and beta-carotene. One jar of BAC nutritionally exceeds twelve trucks of Alfalfa.

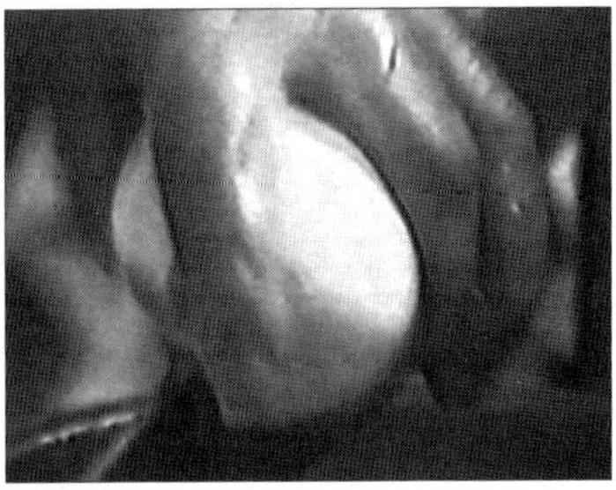

BAC – FED CHICKEN EGGS
Larger and with high concentrations of curative nutrients

It was very rewarding for Mr. Kiriac to see many researchers and project workers "misappropriate" BAC for themselves and their families, friends, and pets. There was a "blind-eye" policy applied to these "white" thefts.

During that period on the poultry farm, significant side research with rabbits was completed, primarily because of certain cancers that were affecting these species in Moldova. Rabbits were excellent research subjects because they reproduce three times a year.

The results were of great importance and a revelation to Mr. Kiriac. The cancers were eradicated in the first year. It was observed that the rabbits with BAC in their diet would bear two to three more offspring. Additionally, their fur was much shinier and longer.

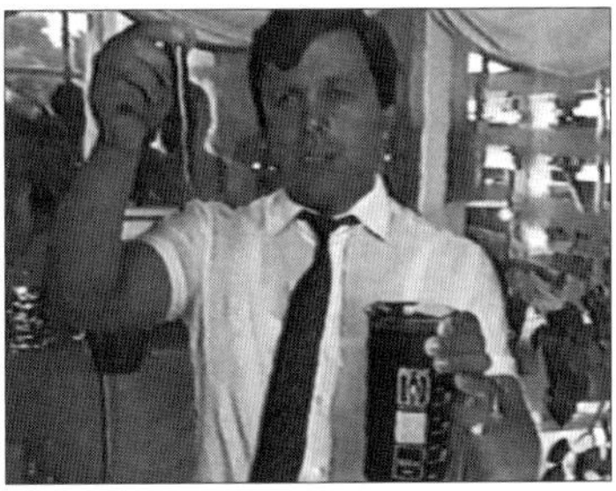

MR. KIRIAC HOLDING BAC IN LAB
One jar of BAC nutritionally exceeds twelve trucks of Alfalfa

The USSR expended hundreds of millions of dollars into the research and application of BAC to livestock. Unfortunately, all of the benefits and results of BAC were slow to be accepted in the USSR. The conservative bodies were lobbied by the pharmaceutical industry or politically influenced in other ways to maintain the established methods of using antibiotics and growth hormones, somewhat like the situation in the USA today.

While Mr. Kiriac was creating marvelous results in Moldova, Mikhail Gorbachev was elected President of the USSR in March of 1985. Under his leadership, great advances took place, even in the wake of a disaster. Mr. Kiriac was now ready to accept one of his greatest challenges in helping people with BAC.

CHERNOBYL NUCLEAR DISASTER AND BAC'S HEALING POWER

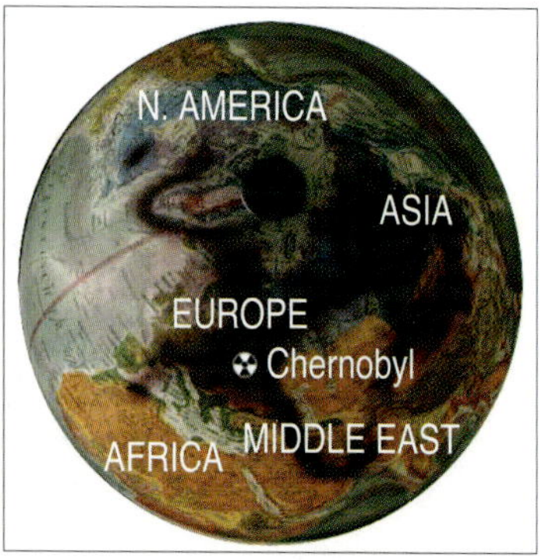

CHERNOBYL RADIATION CLOUD
The dark cloud indicates the extent of the radiation April 27 - May 06, just after the accident in Chernobyl.

The Chernobyl nuclear power plant reactor exploded on April 26th 1986, creating chaos, extreme pain, and suffering, but at the same time allowing major advances in the human application of BAC. The disaster was a major event in the life of Mr. Kiriac and his family, and of course for the USSR at large. War measures were enacted for all of Russia after the explosion and were maintained for months.

The extent of the disaster was increasing everyday and its potential spread remained unknown. Mr. Kiriac and his family lived 500 km (about 300 miles) from the epicenter and were subjected to radiation directly as well as through the local food from plants and animals. Both his children, Rodika and Stefana, were affected like most local children. Both daughters had marks on the head and body. Rodika, then seven, was losing up to two-inch wide patches of hair.

Mr. Kiriac fed BAC to his entire family, putting them on daily rations of the thick paste concentrates, fresh from the bioreactor. To this day, the oldest daughter, Rodika, can still remember the strong smell and taste of BAC. She is very grateful to her father for providing his wonderful invention to the family. Today, both daughters are healthy, beautiful young women.

When disaster struck at Chernobyl, Ukraine, not only was the region around the reactor affected, but the neighboring state of Belarus received 70% of the radioactive fallout and 23% of its territory became contaminated. Over 160,000 children and 146,000 cleanup workers were victims of radiation poisoning which resulted in birth defects, leukemia, cancer, and thyroid disease, degeneration of spinal fluids, liver and bone marrow, as well as anemia, loss of vision and appetite, and a severely compromised immune system.

Because of his previous success with BAC and various cancers in many animal species, and with humans in smaller scale clinical studies, Mr. Kiriac was able to work locally with adults and children from neighborhood schools that were suffering from radiation exposure.

BAC was administered in therapeutic doses, and Mr. Kiriac, working with a small team, was able to closely monitor the regenerative power of BAC. Several health improvements were noted:

- Leukemia, dangerously low white blood cell counts were significantly redressed in less then 20 days, leading to rapid improvements in the health of treated children compared to others who did not receive BAC

- Regeneration of bone marrow, spinal fluids, blood, and liver
- Reduction in urine radioactivity levels by more then 40% in less then 20 days
- Many other virtual miracles were observed

Amazingly, there was health restoration even when children's disease was so advanced that their eyeballs where bulging out of their sockets. In addition, the healing occurred during continuous presence of radiation as well as contaminated food and water sources.

Many people died as a result of the Chernobyl explosion, but the miracles were numerous. Given the super nutrients in BAC, rapid progress in healing was observed and several of the victims treated survived and are alive today.

Mr. Kiriac remarks, "It is important to note that the Chernobyl disaster is still ongoing. Even though the exploded reactor is "sealed" in concrete, radiation continues to escape not only into the local atmosphere, but due to winds, into the world atmosphere as well."

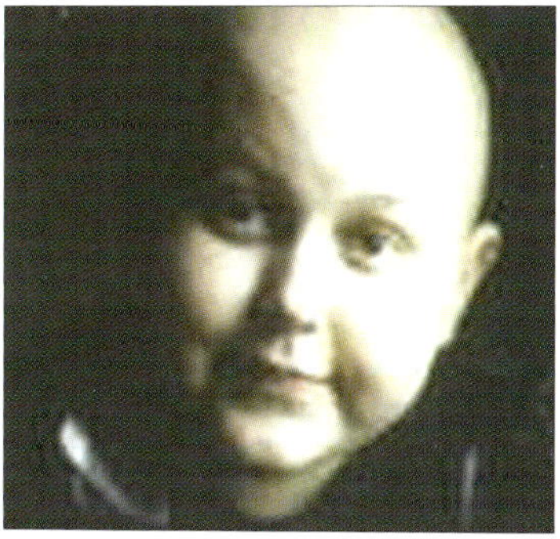

CHERNOBYL CHILD
160,000 children suffered from radiation illnesses. BAC saved many thousands.

MORE PROJECTS ADD TO THE SUCCESS OF BAC

Mr. Kiriac's growing reputation in the nutrition research circles, especially in the Ministry of Science, allowed him the opportunity to become a much respected leader. He was able to influence the formation and to head projects that he felt would be most beneficial to his goal of proving that nutrition is the best healing and health source for animals and humans.

Although the Ministry of Nutrition Science was somewhat influenced by the USSR's medical system, which like the USA system imposes rules such as the use of antibiotics, he stopped short of embracing all their concepts: he did not vaccinate his animal subjects and focused on nutrition as opposed to drugs.

His published papers showed great scientific progress towards his ultimate goals. Had the USSR maintained its strong world presence, Mr. Kiriac's goal could have become a reality: make the USSR a world leader in nutritional solutions to suppress disease and promote health. During this period, the USSR was suffering many threats to its existence: economic, political, and military. The continuation of the research was driven by Mr. Kiriac and supported by the ministries and scientific circles which he was part of.

In 1987, Mr. Kiriac was nominated Moldova's Person of the Year for his resounding achievement and success at the most economically significant poultry center which provided considerable financial return for Moldova. In honor of the occasion, a lengthy documentary was produced and televised on national TV (Note that most of the photos that you see in this booklet were taken from this documentary film).

VORONEZH YIELDS A SECOND BIOREACTOR

An epidemic of various cancers was decimating the pig population around Voronezh area in Russia. Following the resounding success with the poultry industry in Moldova, the prestigious Moscow Academy of Sciences became very interested in the BAC research and results. It was suggested (an order and honor you did not refuse) that Mr. Kiriac join the team in Voronezh to build a second bioreactor and research center, then proceed immediately to stop the local epidemic of cancers with the pig population.

Voronezh was the premier biologic research center and the largest and most influential scientific health center in the former USSR and in all of Europe. Shortly after the arrival of Mr. Kiriac, a bioreactor was built and the exact BAC blends for pigs were developed. Within one year, the epidemic was under control and the cancers subsiding. Remarkable results were obtained with pigs starting with the second generation when applying the hybridizing (cross breeding) of species. There was a general productivity increase with augmentation in the number of newborn per litter, an increase in survival rate from 98% to 99%, genetic health increases transmitted to next generations, and significantly better tasting meats. Similar positive results had been observed with cows, minks, and rabbits. Noticeably, the best results were obtained when working with animals born of parents fed BAC in their feed starting at least 10 to 12 days before conception.

WITH SUCCESS CAME OPPORTUNITY

Following the success at Voronezh, Mr. Kiriac was appointed General Manager at the Moscow Academy of Sciences to further prepare for the next test bed for livestock. Detailed plans were formulated for a first test farm in Lithuania for modeling a broader rollout of biological and livestock production in Russia. Lithuania was the best place politically as it was already receptive to this kind of forward thinking. Lithuania was also quite open to alternative medicine while the rest of the USSR remained more conservative.

However, following the political struggles in the USSR, this was not to happen. The efforts in Moscow included the allopathic model to blend or develop the ideal medication for both human and animals. Mr. Kiriac had to fight many pressures from the allopathic model to maintain his assertions that nutrition was the best solution.

SAVING THE MINKS

In 1989, an epidemic of various cancers was decimating the mink population in Siberia, mostly around the large city of Omsk. The mink industry in the USSR was an important and historically beloved industry because of minks' superior fur. Once again, the Nutrition department of the Moscow Academy of Sciences ordered Mr. Kiriac to join the team in Omsk to eliminate the cancers and save the industry.

The first order was to build a local bioreactor, providing BAC for the project as well as for the region in the future. The effort proceeded to fine-tune the right BAC concentrate blends for minks and to add them to their diet.

By the following year, the epidemic was under control and the cancers subsided. This was further evidence of the power of BAC, which created greater support for Mr. Kiriac, who was by now respected for his research and success.

SIBERIA'S VOLCANIC WATERS YIELD HOT DISCOVERIES

As a result of political changes beginning in 1989, the USSR rapidly disassembled in a short period causing major economic, political, and geographical changes for the entire region. Mr. Kiriac was looking forward to the breakdown of the Berlin wall and of the communist system, as were most of his countrymen. Without the impediment of the USSR central government's bureaucracy, he envisioned a strong democratic economy in which they would be able to rapidly promote the concepts of BAC: socialistically to help people and commercially for the livestock industry.

Contrary to his hopes, the breakdown of the USSR brought out more endemic social problems of alcoholism, general apathy, and laziness, resulting from the many years under a communist regime. Worse yet, this allowed for organized crime to reign. All these factors greatly affected the budgets for BAC research and the launch of algae and organic farming. Moldova regained its independence, but was left with significant economic hurdles and problems.

Nevertheless, the next year, as part of the continued research projects, Mr. Kiriac made the proposal to create a BAC bioreactor on the volcanic peninsula of Kamchatka, Siberia. Despite the bureaucratic and controlling rules in place at the time in Russia, this project was pushed through and approved within one week. Even under budget constraints in post-USSR Russia, Mr. Kiriac was able to obtain continued support in subsequent years.

The Kamchatka bioreactor was built in the next four months and proved to deliver more than what Mr. Kiriac had expected. He had selected this specific location because of the presence of extraordinary volcanic nutrients in the water. This ideal water contained 92 and more trace elements, including selenium and sodium bicarbonate, all naturally occurring in an ideal temperature of 35° to 37° C (95° to 99° F). This was a perfect base solution for BAC and allowed the presence of the best Essential Fatty Acids (EFA's) within BAC, some of them yet unknown to science.

ACCOLADES PRELUDE DRAMATIC CHANGES

In 1990, Michael Kiriac received his Doctorate in Biotechnology. He was assigned to the Department of Nutrition at the Moscow Nutrition Sciences Research Institute while continuing to supervise all of his ongoing research.

Three years later, as a further verification of BAC and his work at Chernobyl, the Belarus Ministry of Health concluded: "algae preparations decrease radiation dose load received from food contaminated with radionucleides, Cesium-137 and Strontium-90, and promote the evacuation of radionuclide's from the human body." No side effects were ever registered.

In spite of this, it was becoming apparent that to continue his work, Dr. Kiriac would have to leave Russia. His homeland, Moldova, had become very poor and still is – the industrial enterprises had broken down. It was very difficult to be a scientist, and being an entrepreneur at heart, working in the current system was next to impossible. His imminent decision to leave was clear, however, the transition to a new country would prove to be difficult.

NORTH AMERICA – STRESS AND OPPORTUNITY

In 1995, Dr. Kiriac presented his invention at a conference in Brussels, Belgium. It was there that he met a Canadian diplomat suffering from diabetes, for whom Dr. Kiriac provided BAC. After talking about the conditions in Moldova and hearing about Canada, Dr. Kiriac accepted an offer for assistance in preparing and facilitating immigration documents for all of his family to move to Canada.

This was a very difficult decision for him and his family, but he believed that with his Doctorate as well as with his scientific expertise and knowledge, he would be able to easily transition his business into Canada.

NOT THE DREAMLAND EXPECTED

So, the following year, he moved to Montreal with his wife Liudmila and daughters Rodika, 17, and Stefana, 11. Contrary to his hope, the transition to Canada was much more stressful and sobering than anticipated. Their first realization was that learning Quebec's two languages – French and English – would take at least a year, and this would slow up his ability to open his business and earn a living. In addition, finding work was not as easy as expected – Quebec had a high unemployment rate at the time and the competition was fierce. Before he could establish his business, he had to work for other providers of health products and solutions.

Compounding his problems, coming to Canada he had left not only his birth family and his homeland – he had left all his support systems. In retrospect, he could have immigrated to Europe as the European scientific community had already recognized his work and continues to do so with accolades and awards. European companies did and continue to pursue him to join them because of his scientific research and success.

In addition, the Canadian mainstream medical model, patterned after the UK and the USA, did not honor his naturopathic work. In fact, the tendency was to suppress it since it ran counter to the concepts of drugs and surgery as the solution to disease and health conditions.

Regardless, he managed to quickly learn how the Canadian capitalist system functions well enough to be back in production in three years.

MORE TRAGEDY DEMANDS PRODUCTION FACILITY

While working towards his goal, in 1997, his oldest sister, friend and second mother, Eugenia, was diagnosed with pancreatic cancer at the age of 71. Dr. Kiriac was still struggling, so he had neither the money nor the equipment to formulate the BAC recipe which he already knew would save his beloved sister – nor was he in a position to contact Ukraine to assist with her treatment. Upon her death, he was devastated – the pain and frustration were enormous. At the same time, his wife began to suffer severe anemia from the stress of the earlier radiation effects of Chernobyl, the relocation away from close family, and the life change. The condition was very severe.

He resolved to accelerate production of BAC in Canada. In addition to his sister's death and his wife's condition, Dr. Kiriac became very concerned with the significant levels of diseases in America at large. Diseases that he was not accustomed to seeing in Eastern Europe included: diabetics, obesity, Alzheimer's disease, a high occurrence of heart and cardiovascular problems, and cancers of many sorts.

Dr. Kiriac attributes these diseases to the poor nutrition habits in our countries, to the high and uncontrolled stress in our lives, the high levels of pollution in the air, and to the processes our foods are subjected to: preservatives, additives, canning, and overcooking. Sugar, alcohol, drugs, and fast foods are terrible addictions for the vast majority of Canadians and Americans. Contributing to these problems, there is a significant abuse and misuse of medication and supplements.

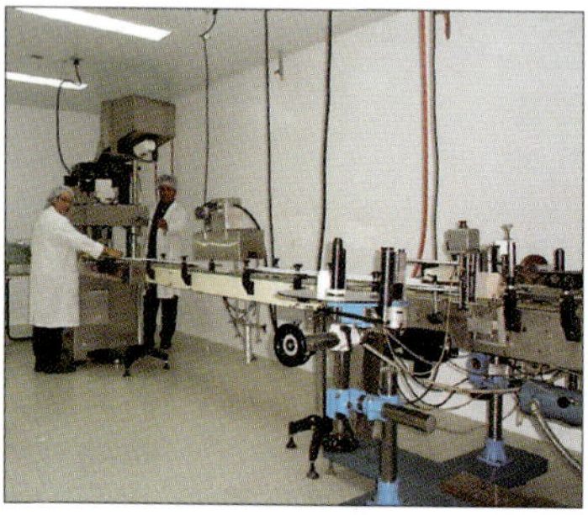

PROCESSING PLANT
Latest technologies, invented by Dr. Kiriac, are applied today in the manufacturing and processing cycles of BAC. For example, the encapsulating and bottling plant is equipped with ultra-violet lighting which kills airborne bacteria, assuring a clean and safe product.

Later in 1997, Dr. Kiriac brought BAC alive in Canada to help people with these health problems. He founded BioNutrition to begin formulating BAC products. But the harsh realities of life were to delay his plans. Besides the significant investments required setting up the production, Dr. Kiriac was still in a steep learning curve with the French and English languages, and had to have other employments to survive economically.

Two years later, Dr. Kiriac realized his dream and began distributing BAC in Canada. The algae are still grown and harvested in the world's richest volcanic peninsula of Kamchatka, Russia and then imported to Canada for blending, encapsulating, and bottling under strict quality assurance. He remains a pioneer in the industry and continues to consult other growers about advanced alga-growing technologies, which he invented.

His wife, Liudmila, has been taking BAC and is in excellent health ever since.

NORTH AMERICAN VALIDATION OF BAC

Very soon after his arrival in Canada, Dr. Kiriac came to realize that all of his work and research done in a country far away would not cut it in North America. He knew that he would have to re-prove his work locally in ways that would be credible to the livestock industry and eventually to the people. As Dr. Kiriac soon discovered, in America it is easier to market a new product for people then it is for the animal industry, which is more rigidly guarded.

I remember early on, when in an effort to help the cause, I would suggest to Dr. Kiriac to conduct small research projects, he would respond each time in the same way: “Roland, the research is done, this concept, this product, is proven already”. Yet he knew that he would have to conduct small and maybe larger trials in America to gain the trust of the industry and the people. Being a man of action, he started on this quest to make BAC a reality in America.

THE MCGILL UNIVERSITY POULTRY STUDY

From 1999 to 2000, working with the research department of the Montreal McGill University, Dr. Kiriac initiated the first of several small scale trials to take place in America. He was able to reproduce on a much smaller scale the poultry productivity results achieved in Moldova. Out of the two test groups of 13,000 chickens each, the group with BAC added to their grain demonstrated the expected results over the group not fed BAC: larger eggs, stronger shells, more eggs per month, reduction of bad fat, and reduction in the birth mortality rate. The test was performed twice for accuracy. The following graphs show two clear results with the group taking BAC when compared with the standard group not on BAC.

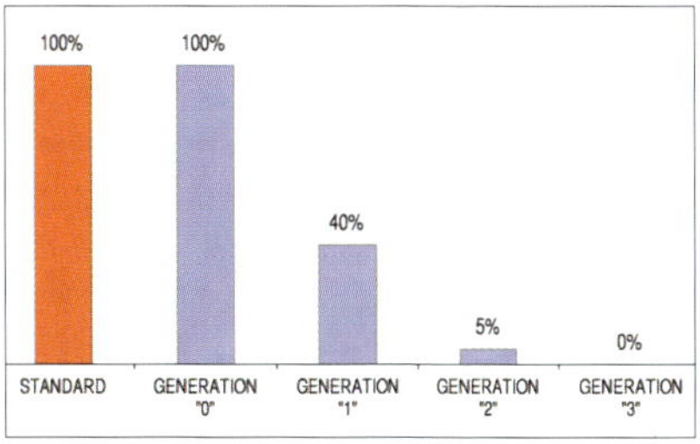

REDUCTION IN FAT CONTENT

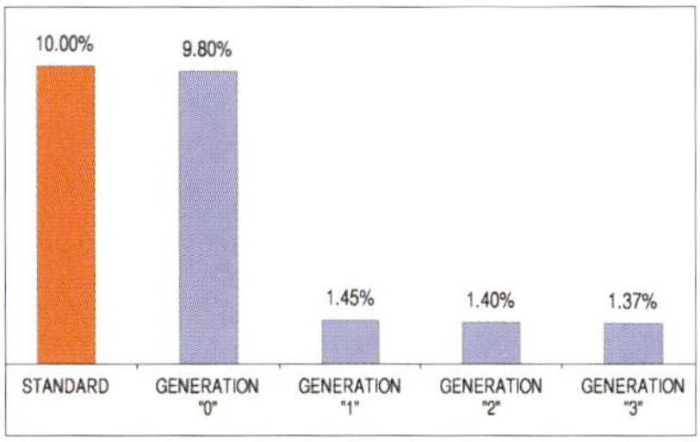

REDUCTION IN BIRTH MORTALITY

THE ALAIN FORGET DAIRY FARM

In January of 2004, an agreement was reached with Alain Forget, the owner and manager of the "Alain Forget Dairy Farm" located in Laval, Quebec, to evaluate BAC in regards to a set of productivity markers for 22 dairy cows part of a herd of 50 Holstein cows. BAC is incorporated into the commercial feeds that are fed daily to the cows with the purpose of increasing productivity.

At the start of the evaluation, the herd was already performing above average, but for the purpose of this evaluation, certain parameters were targeted for amelioration: milk volume, texture of the udder, somatic cell count (SCC), overall productivity, emptying of the udder, gestation period, and reduction of nervousness of the cow during milking which may lead to greater emptying of the udder. The results of this ongoing evaluation are monitored at regular intervals by Valacta, an independent provincial dairy center of expertise regulated by the Quebec Dairy Industry.

Prior to the following report, three reports had been provided by Alain Forget at intervals of 6 months, 12 months, and 24 months. These reports can be made available to the reader upon request or by visiting our website (see inside front cover). Following is the summary of the results after 36 months of evaluation as written by Alain Forget in August of 2008.

"For 36 months we have been using bio-algae concentrates with a group of cows within our Holstein dairy herd. The results show a 3,000 kg augmentation of milk production over 36 months, a general augmentation of the Breed Class Average (BCA) of 20% for milk, 9.3% in fat, and 8.6% in protein. These results have earned us the General Herd Performance award from Valacta, the Quebec milk control agency. We have also observed the following results when compared to provincial averages; a gestation interval of 384 days as compared to 426 for the provincial average; a milk production of 12,186 kg per year compared to 8,622 kg; a 434 kg production of fat versus a provincial average of 329 kg; and a protein production of 399 kg as opposed to 278 kg for provincial.

During this period, the evaluated herd increased from 22 cows to 40 lactating cows. The augmentation of the average age of the herd has an influence on the somatic cell count (SCC). We observed our SCC distorted by nearly 34% because of two or three cows. With the deviation, the count stands at 235,000, slightly over the provincial average. During the months of March to May, the SCC stood below the provincial average of 110,000, with 105,000 in March, 102,000 in April, and 65,000 in May. Because of the independently and statistically measured results obtained with our herd, we believe that BAC must affect positively the brain organ hypothalamus, which is responsible for the metabolism regulation. We are excited to continue the evaluation with focus on a healthier udder, longevity of the herd, and thus increased profits for the farm."

Alain Forget, President, Alain Forget Dairy Farm
Laval, Quebec, Canada, August 2008

The following table shows the Breed Class Average (BCA) data collected at the different intervals during the evaluation.

	MILK	FAT	PROTEINS
PRE-TEST	10 039 kgs	219 kgs	223 kgs
6 MONTHS	10 565 kgs	242 kgs	236 kgs
12 MONTHS	10 439 kgs	228 kgs	227 kgs
24 MONTHS	12 039 kgs	239 kgs	242 kgs
36 MONTHS	13 039 kgs	239 kgs	242 kgs
DIFFERENCE	3 000 kgs	20 kgs	19 kgs
IMPROVEMENT	29.9%	9.1%	8.5%

IMPROVEMENT IN MILK, FAT, AND PROTEIN

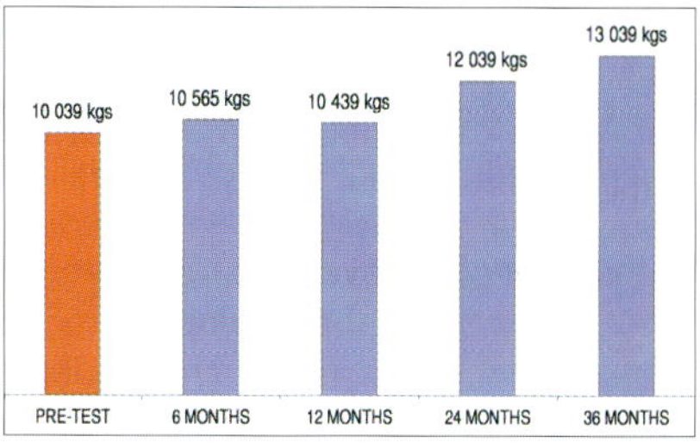

MILK PRODUCTION

In the province of Quebec, Valacta maintains several provincial productivity measurements and their statistics and Alain Forget's results are shown next alongside provincial averages for Quebec.

	PROVINCIAL	ALAIN FORGET	DIFFERENCE
LONGEVITY	39 days	42 days	3 days
PROTEINS	278 kgs	399 kgs	121 kgs
FAT	329 kgs	434 kgs	105 kgs
GESTATION	426 days	384 days	- 42 days
MILK PRODUCTION	8 622 kgs	12 186 kgs	3 564 kgs

COMPARISON OF QUEBEC PROVINCIAL DATA WITH ALAIN FORGET'S RESULTS

When working with animals in testing dietary changes for health or productivity, there are no placebo affects, and it is much easier to ensure that all participants are eating the same diet; thus the results can be significantly more valid than those from the tests with humans. Based on the verified increase in many productivity factors for the 22 cows in this study, we must conclude that BAC augments cellular nutrition to the brain hypothalamus-pituitary axis which regulates the metabolism and brings about a positive impact on the endocrine and central nervous systems.

SAVING MERRI MASON'S BIGHORN SHEEP

In October 2007 we began a study in cooperation with Merri Mason, owner of a herd of bighorn sheep that were more or less destined to die from Johne's disease. Usually this disease kills most animals of the herd by the time they reach 2 years of age. Johne's disease (pronounced "yo-knees") is a contagious, chronic, and often fatal infection that affects primarily the small intestine of ruminants. It is caused by a bacterium called Mycobacterium avium subspecies paratuberculosis. Johne's disease has been reported all around the world in cattle for several decades. Although it has also been reported in sheep for many years, no one is certain of how widespread it is or exactly how much damage it is doing to our sheep industry. BAC is added to the daily feed of 12 bighorn sheep's selected amongst the herd of 35 that are affected by Johne's disease with the purpose of saving the sheep by increasing their overall cellular nutrition, vitality, and immunity. For the purpose of the study the selected sheep are kept apart from the main herd. At the start of evaluation, the herd was already being decimated by Johne's and the owner was thinking of euthanizing the entire herd as recommended by the veterinarian. Often once a herd is affected, there is no other solution. Read following Merri's report after 11 months of testing.

"Well finally had a chance to get together this brief testimonial on the effects of BAC on my bighorn sheep. First, I want you to know that I have not had a symptomatic sheep in 9 months. The two rams that were born with symptoms, although undersized, appear to be fine. What first comes to mind is the hair quality. All the lambs on the program from conception have superior hair coats from the last crop. The hair is softer and shinier. The color seems to be intensified as well. I also notice them to be calmer and easier to wean. Horn growth on the 2-3 month old rams comes sooner and with bigger diameter at the base and length overall for that age. Now we know that the symptoms of the disease usually shows up at or just after age two, so we will have to wait on these rams awhile. BUT I have quite a few sheep that have passed their two year birthdays that did not get the algae until they were over a year that seem symptom free. Another interesting factor is that I have two sheep from the original herd that are at least 4 years old, and appear symptom free. Many of the sheep from that herd died from the disease. It seems that there are so many factors to consider with Johne's. Some are symptomatic, some carriers with no symptoms, etc. I believe the best test will be the two young rams that were born with symptoms, and now appear symptom free. We will be closer to the truth when they are two.

I think this is a good place to start, because the rams that started on your product a year ago are starting to turn two years. All of the sheep coats are thick and colors are intensified. I have also noticed a calmer nature and ease of handling with these normally difficult to handle breeds. During gestation the ewes seem to gain weight almost too rapidly. I often have to cut back on the dosage during this time and lactation or the ewes get too fat and produce too much milk. I no longer have the problem of a ewe's drastic weight loss due to feeding twins over a three month period. I have also reduced the amount of grain I feed with the same results as the former amount.

So far all are healthy, but the most amazing thing is their horns. I have enclosed photos of Ramsey and Gunner – they have the horn growth of three to four year old rams at barely two years. These rams and the crop behind them also have larger body mass than previous crops with the same bloodline.

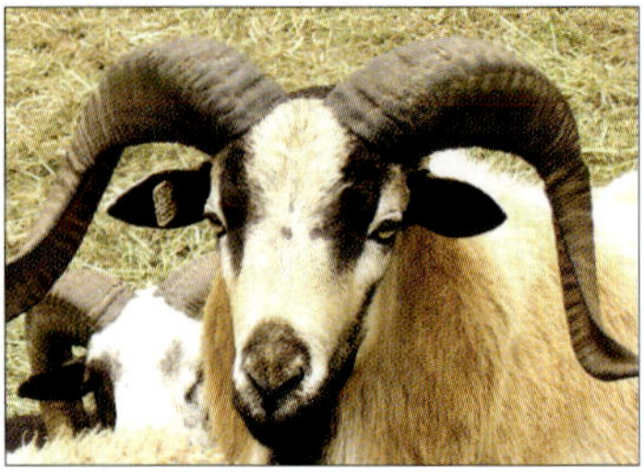

RAMSEY

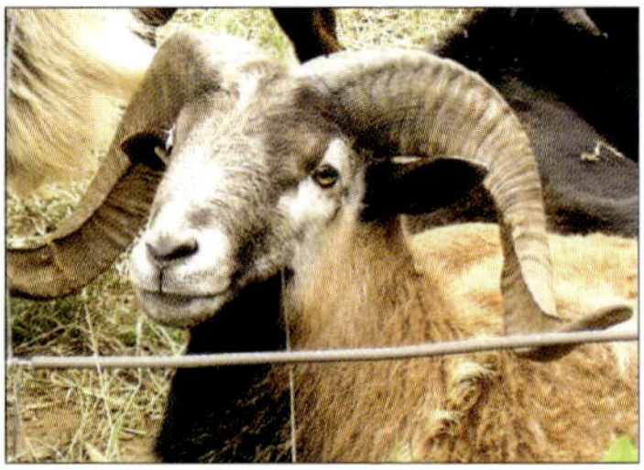

GUNNER

Humpfrey and Jackson, two rams born sick out of the sick ewes that died within weeks of delivering are undersized for their age, but are symptom free at this time.

They will be a year old in November. They both got a bad start because they were undernourished during development, and the brown one had poor quality milk from the ewe. Humpfrey is a real stinker, hates to be caught, and gets out of everything true to his Mouflon nature. Jackson is totally tame much like a cat. He also likes to ram the cats and steal their food. I feel totally blessed that you both have given me the opportunity to save my herd and demonstrate the benefits of your product. I have actually started thinking that I could sell some of my sheep again without wondering if I am causing grief in someone else's herd. The frustration I have experienced with turning buyers and breeders away after working on the breeding aspects of this herd for 4 years is difficult to describe. You and the Doctor have given me some hope that at least I can keep my beautiful animals and not have to helplessly watch them die."

Merri Mason, Owner, Bighorn Sheep Farm, Ohio, USA - October 2008

At this point in the study, it appears that the goal to save Merri's sheep, including some of those already infected before the study began, and certainly their offspring's, may very well be achieved. Meanwhile, the many benefits (underlined in Merri's letter) observed to date with the sheep, are much of the same that were obtained during the Russian research with several species: calmer mood, shinier hair and coat, larger healthier animal, less feed needed, increased survival rate, prevention of mad cow disease, prevention of various viral and bacterial infections, healthier animal from one generation to the next, prevention of osteoporosis and increase in bone mass, increased fertility, increased protein and good fats in milk, eggs and meat, and many more.

Dr. Michael Kiriac had never worked with bighorn sheep and when asked about the success observed so far, he commented: *"When the animal eats BAC which feeds the brain efficiently, the brain organs awaken. The hypothalamus alone is responsible for homeostasis of all body metabolisms, including that of energy. With BAC all metabolisms awaken; assimilation and absorption of nutrients from foods improves, such as protein assimilation and absorption (hence less feed is needed for the sheep), mineral metabolisms, synthesis of proteins and enzymes within cells. When Collagen metabolism becomes more efficient (Collagen is the main protein of connective tissue in animals and the most abundant protein in mammals, making up about 25% to 35% of the whole-body protein content), then there is better growth of the animal and stronger and larger horns. In chickens it was larger and stronger eggs; in dairy cows, it was more and better milk with increases in protein and butter fat; in pigs and minks – larger litter; etc."*

WHAT PETS ARE SAYING

For over 8 years BAC has been used with thousands of pets and animal companions in America, with success for most. People are using BAC with their pets for prevention of health issues, and in many cases, for alleviating degenerative conditions of all sorts.

MACINTOSH BEATS THE CANCER ODDS

"Macintosh (Cairn Terrier, 10 years, 23 lbs) was diagnosed with hemangiosarcoma and had surgery to remove the cancer tumor and spleen. He was given an estimate of 6 months to live (if lucky) after surgery. He is getting BAC and is enjoying life now, more than 36 months (as of Nov 2007) after the procedure and still doing well. Thank you for helping Macintosh beat the cancer odds and giving him a new lease on life." - N.A., USA

CHRONIC RENAL FAILURE

"My 17 year old cat, Brindee was diagnosed with CRF in March. Her BUN was 48, Creatinnine Clearance 4.0. While researching treatment options I found BAC and ordered it immediately. Within a week, Brindee had more appetite, energy and was more social than she's been in years! Two months later her Bun was down to 42, Creatinnine Clearance down to 3.4! My vet was very surprised to say the least. That's when I told him about BAC. I'm documenting Brindee's progress." - T.C., USA

I WAS TOLD TO PUT MY DOG OUT

"I was told to put my dog out, that it had a few weeks to live. With natural food, bottled water and the Bio-Algae Concentrates, my giant Schnauzer had 10 additional months of comfortable and happy life. Thank you for all your help." - Thor B., Virginia, USA.

SWELLED LYMPH NODES

"My dog Harley was diagnosed with Lymphoma Sarcoma in February 2004. My naturopathic vet recommended your product, though he had not yet used it in his practice. I ordered BAC and started giving it to him daily. His lymph nodes "disappeared" (shrunk to normal) within 2 weeks..." - Kim B, Seattle, Washington, USA – June 2004

WHAT PEOPLE ARE SAYING

For over 8 years BAC has been used by people in America, with success for most. People are using BAC for prevention of health issues, and in many cases, for alleviating degenerative conditions of all sorts. I am relating a few cases below.

LEUKEMIA

"I just wanted to share with you some great news. I got my mother in law on BAC because she has leukemia. Her doctor wanted to put her on all this medicine for her rising cholesterol and white blood cells. She told him to wait one month and she would get blood work again and they could go from there. Just after one month with BAC (she didn't change anything else) her levels all dropped.

- *Total cholesterol 258 to 185!*
- *Triglycerides 223 to 135!*
- *Bad cholesterol 163 to 112!*
- *White cell count went back to normal!*

The doctor asked her what meds he put her on, thinking he forgot to write it in her chart. Smiling back she said "none", and proceeded to tell him about the supplement. He just rolled up his eyes, even after seeing her results in the blood work! Go figure, maybe some day he'll choose to look into it for his clients. I just wanted to thank you for such an amazing product. It has also helped tremendously with my Newfoundland who has kidney disease. Thanks" - Shannon, Paws & Claws, Breckenridge, Colorado, USA

EPILEPSY

Brenda, a 32 years old woman from California, USA, shared her experience of using BAC as follows: *"I have had no seizures in 10 months - I have suffered from epileptic seizures since I was a child. When taking medication I would get seizure 3 to 4 times per week. Without medication I could get them daily. With BAC and without medication I have not had one seizure since the first day I started taking bio-algae concentrates six months ago now. Because of my success I recently gave some BAC to my cousin and he has not had a seizure in seven weeks".*

When Brenda related her continuing success with BAC, I was curious and I asked Dr. Kiriac about the mechanisms of action between BAC and Brenda's amazing results. As usual his answer was humble. He said:

"Roland, we don't know much about brain diseases. We know there are billions of brain cells and synapses and on/off electrical connections and requirement for nutrients and resulting cellular energy, growth, protection and regeneration. We know there are parts of the brain that regulate rational thoughts and others that regulate basic motor controls. We know that certain areas of the brain are more likely than others to be involved in seizure activity. The motor cortex, which is responsible for body movement, and the temporal lobes, including the hippocampus, which is involved in memory, are particularly sensitive to biochemical changes (e.g., decreased oxygen level, metabolic imbalances, infection) that provoke abnormal brain cell activity.

The greatest value of using BAC is its direct influence on the hypothalamus / pituitary relationship. This glandular cortex is responsible for all metabolic activities in our body. When this life critical cortex is properly nourished and energized, it holds the power to command the body metabolisms back to balance and health via a myriad of hormones and peptides. For example, one important metabolism is the nutrients to energy conversion (Krebs cycle/ATP) for which the balance in salt/sodium, potassium, magnesium and calcium is critical. This electrical and atomic energy generation occurs unceasingly in each mitochondrion of every trillion cells of our body including those at the root of epileptic seizures".

We have since witnessed new success with BAC and epilepsy in children and adults. BAC is a food that's easy to use and is non-toxic; there are no known contra-indications and no negative side effects.

HIV

In February 2004, a Boulder, Colorado MD reported to me Daniel's case and suggested we followed his progress together. Daniel had been diagnosed HIV positive years earlier and was seeing his condition worsening alarmingly. Following our recommendations to use BAC and to change his eating habits, Daniel saw his viral load drop significantly in a few weeks. Let me show you a perspective of continued progress in his words:

"I am HIV positive. I just got my latest lab work back and it's great! My viral load is stable at about 10,000 (the nurse practitioner said she was very surprised just how stable that it is), and my T-cells are up over 400! That's the highest they've been in over a year. If you will recall, exactly one year ago my viral load was at 139,000 and the T-cells barely over 250, prompting the docs to want to start me on meds. But then I started the BAC. I am especially impressed with the numbers because since October, when I returned from Brazil, I've been dealing with some very difficult emotions like grief, sadness, and some depression. There has been a lot of stress as I've tried to find a job (still looking). Also, I haven't been very strict nutritionally as that has been difficult as well. Given these factors, I'm so thrilled that my numbers are so good. It gives me new energy and motivation to eat right, and continue trying to make good lifestyle choices. But I think if it weren't for the bio-algae concentrates, the picture would look very different right now. Thank you!"
- Daniel - February 2005, USA

Following another test in May 2006, Daniel sent this note:

"My latest results show a drop in viral load to just over 5,000. My CD4s are stable at 414. Interestingly, my numbers continue to look good despite huge amounts of stress at my work. But I continue to take the BAC and the numbers are either stable or have actually improved".

At the time when this edition was published, Daniel has continued to keep the disease in check without medications and their side effects, without long term liver damage, and only with a few capsules of BAC per day. As commented by Daniel, he is doing well, even if under a lot of stress and without being "perfect" with his diet.

LYME DISEASE

"I have been very ill for 4 years. I was bit by a tick carrying Ehrlichia and Lyme disease. Unknown to me at the time, the head of the tick was left in my side. Four months later, I was bitten several times by a Brown Recluse Spider. Between the two bites I got very ill, bedridden for 4 weeks, and with a massive medical intervention. I almost died. For one year, I suffered with severe joint and muscle pain and headaches. I was often weak and couldn't get comfortable in any position. I started taking BAC and within a few weeks of starting a friend that knew of my condition who had not seen me in a while asked me what I was doing because she said I looked great. Well, I thought about it and realized I had been feeling better and the only change that I had made was that I had been taking BAC. I am a true believer that BAC has brought me back to a healthy functioning person." - Robin H.

GLAUCOMA AND OSTEOPOROSIS

"My pressure for the Glaucoma continues to be good. As well, my bone density had improved so much over the space of a year that my doctor could not believe the readings! I am still taking nine capsules daily and trying to space them at one and a half hour intervals." - Gail, USA

ENERGY, STAMINA, AND MOOD

"Instead of the usual 2 pm slump I experienced in the afternoon, my energy level is maintained throughout the day. I feel well-fed on this product. My body feels nourished." - M. Bennett, USA

KIDNEY FUNCTION IMPROVED TO 24%

"Now kidney function is up to 24%, a 6% increase over the last twelve months. I feel certain BAC is the reason. I have been taking BAC for over a year now. My diet otherwise is awful. I have been eating one meal every other day. I like that and hope for more improvement since the prognosis a year ago was only eventual dialysis." - F&BB, CA, USA

NO NEED FOR SURGERY

"I was a lineman for the local power company for many years and suffered with very painful knees most of that time. My doctor said I would have to have both knees replaced, which I wasn't looking forward to, so I put it off. A couple years ago a friend introduced me to BAC, and after taking it for only a few weeks, I had absolutely no pain and there was no need for any surgery. I am completely retired now at 74 but very active and busy gardening and mowing lawns for people. I also clear snow in the winter with no pain whatsoever." G. Fenske, Wisconsin, USA

SPORTS AND ATHLETICS

During the 2000 Winter Games held in St. Petersburg Russia, BAC was compared with two other supplements – Ginseng and a Chinese herb. It was reported as best by the Russian hockey team for general pain reduction, particularly knee pains as well as faster and better recuperation of energy and blood oxidation after games.

Igor Kravcuk and Pavel Bure, team members and NHL players, sponsored the test and carried BAC to the team in Russia, as well as reported this success to Dr. Kiriac in Montreal.

INTERNATIONAL WRESTLING CHAMPION

"I have been taking this supplement now for a while, I started training three weeks ago and the improvements that I make are just insane. I take three in the morning and three in the afternoon and my friends, who are professional fighters, all ask me what I am using. Strength-wise and endurance-wise I am making crazy improvements. My neighbor is 56 years old, he used to be Stallone's bodyguard for 17 years, and he's taking it too and can't believe what he's doing right now, training hard and recovering like crazy. I truly believe that it can be only because of the BAC, since that's the only thing I use. Everywhere I come people ask me what my training routine is, when I tell them that I started training three weeks ago after a 14 month layoff, they don't believe me. Many will think for sure that I am doing something illegal, like steroids, but trust me, that stuff I don't use, they can actually test me with ANY test they want, and if they want to put their money where their mouth is, I will be happy that bet right away, I can always use some extra cash! Try it out and see how it works for you, what do you have to lose right? Godspeed!"
– Bas Rutten – three times Undefeated King of Pancrase (Hybrid Wrestling), California, USA

GREAT ADJUNCT TO CHIROPRACTIC

"Personally, I have more endurance, I look and feel younger and my hair isn't falling out anymore. I used to see a great deal of hair in the drain prior to taking BAC, but now there is none. At a recent gathering I was told by a woman I have not seen in 5 years that I look so much younger than when we last met. She asked what I was doing and I explained that I started taking BAC a year ago; she was so impressed that she is now a BAC user as well.

Clinically, BAC is a great adjunct to my chiropractic that I never had before. BAC supplies the necessary minerals and proteins to repair the ligaments and as a result, the adjustments hold better.

I also use BAC for women that are looking for hormone replacements as it balances the bodies chemistry and nourishes the nervous system. As a result, hormones become more balanced, hot flashes either diminish or are eliminated and moods become more balanced. The nervous system requires a high-quality protein as the nerves contain mostly protein. Biologically, vegetable protein is more effective than animal protein. The word protein - means first. Every tissue and fluid in the body has protein in it except bile; we need protein to make enzymes. Protein is sloughed off in the skin and nails. The vegetable protein in BAC is complete protein and maintains healthy tissue, feeds the red and white blood cells.

BAC covers so many things: redresses hormone levels, pH and sugar levels, helps the body make enzymes, is a regenerative food."

– Dr. William Johnson, DC, ND, Co-Director of the International Clinic of Biological Cellular Regeneration, Illinois, USA

AWAKENING THE GENIUS WITHIN

In 1999 when I met Michael Kiriac, he told me that consuming BAC was a vastly different concept then that of supplementation. He said that BAC was a "Complement" rather than a "Supplement". He explained that BAC complements the whole rather than supplements a symptom. That got my attention as in those days, as part of my personal health regimen, I was taking more than 20 different supplements daily.

He told me "BAC Awakens the Genius Within". He explained that BAC, due to its completeness, balance, synergies, and bioavailability, is an "extremely" efficient food and that its thousands of nutrients easily reach and nourish the cells of certain areas of the brain that are more difficult to reach than others. By "Genius" he referred specifically to the region of the brain that houses the mission critical "governing" organs of our metabolic health; namely the thalamus, hypothalamus, pituitary and pineal glands, and somewhat the cerebellum.

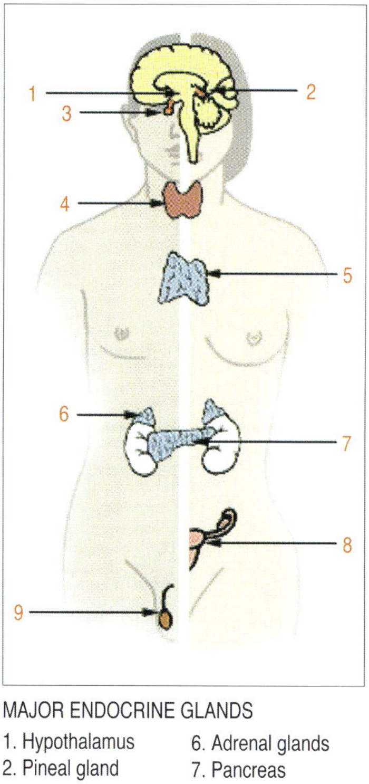

MAJOR ENDOCRINE GLANDS

1. Hypothalamus
2. Pineal gland
3. Pituitary gland
4. Thyroid
5. Thymus
6. Adrenal glands
7. Pancreas
8. Ovaries
9. Testes

Ultimately these organs and glands are responsible for regulating all physiological metabolisms, including energy. These metabolisms include the endocrine system, the sympathetic and Para-sympathetic nervous system, the central nervous system, the lymphatic system, the cardiovascular system, and the digestive system with its critical assimilation, absorption, and elimination functions. In this book I do not write "scientifically" with long winded descriptions of metabolisms or body parts and hundreds of references intended to prove each mechanism of action. As far as I am concerned, the holistic concepts and views of health expressed in this book are scientifically valid and proven by the results obtained with millions of animals as described previously. In line with keeping this book readable, I will refer to this "governing" region of the brain as the "Genius".

The Genius is generally located in the middle and base of the brain. The main function of the Genius is homeostasis, endocrine and energetic coherence, and maintaining the body's status quo. Factors such as energy, blood pressure, body temperature, fluid and electrolyte balance, fat metabolism, and body weight are held to a precise value called the set-points. The Genius and its allies – "the endocrine glands" – are so important that they are called "the guardians of health". In essence, all metabolic functions report back to and are governed by the Genius.

PROBLEMS WITH THE GENIUS

The Genius, like any other part of the body, is comprised of billions of cells, each having a task of its own survival and a specific role. Logically, when the cells that makeup the Genius are healthy and doing their work, then the Genius will perform its overseer role adequately. By deduction, it stands that when the cells that make up the Genius are not healthy and not doing their work, then the Genius will not perform its overseer role adequately.

In order to be healthy and perform their work well, cells need hundreds of nutrients required daily. Only when these nutrients and their energy giving material are supplied will the cells grow, repair, defend from attacks, and perform their specialized metabolic functions.

Because of protective barriers to the brain, the Genius and its billions of cells are more difficult to reach and nourish adequately than the cells in other parts of the body. With aging or disease, the task of nourishing these cells becomes even more difficult and we become less efficient at assimilating nutrients from our foods. This problem is initiated by poor choice of foods, by deficiencies in our diet, and by other intoxicating stressors. Often it is compounded because our foods are depleted of nutrients and/or inassimilable. These problems are sometimes present at birth due to genetics, lifestyle and deficiencies, or they might manifest early during infancy due to poor nutrition.

OPTIMUM CELLULAR FOOD FOR OPTIMUM CELLULAR NUTRITION

Michael Kiriac told me that BAC is an extremely efficient food that results in optimum cellular health. In our various talks, he always brought health to the cellular level. He suggests that there is only one disease – cellular disease, and one health – cellular health.

ONE disease – CELLULAR disease
ONE health – CELLULAR health

In a "purist" holistic perspective, disease (non-health) can be demystified when you work with the cellular level. Let's be realistic; disease and their symptoms reside first at the cellular level. Let's even be scientific; after all, we are made up of hundreds of trillions of intelligent living cells which in turn make up our organs, bones, tissues, blood, and brain. In this model, unhealthy cells lead to unhealthy organs, unhealthy organs lead to deficient metabolic activities, and this in turn leads to symptoms, to which we give a disease name. It is safe to say that once you are diagnosed with a disease that the problem is systemic and its causes have been manifesting in every cell of the body for some time. We don't catch diseases, we make them over time. In the true scientific view, disease is at the cellular level. Let me describe cellular disease in four points:

1. Once symptoms of disease are manifesting (as in hypoglycemia, cholesterol, or high blood pressure), most cells of the body are likely toxic, deficient in nutrients and energy, and are likely less efficient in conducting their myriad of survival activities: repair, detoxification, growth and re-generation, and their specialized contribution as in "insulin" production of certain pancreatic cells.

2. At the next level, due to those cellular deficiencies, the organs are now less efficient in conducting their own metabolic function. For example, with hypoglycemia, we say that the pancreas is sluggish in regulating the blood sugar with adequate insulin.

3. Realize now, that the Genius which is also made of cells, is itself affected by these same cellular deficiencies and is rendered less efficient at regulating metabolisms, like that of blood sugar, pH (acidity/alkalinity), and even the heart beat. You've got a serious problem when the Genius itself is atrophied.

4. Aggravating the problem, after years and decades of metabolic inefficiencies (improper pH, blood sugar, temperature, fats, etc.), the Genius and its allies – the endocrine glands – have become tolerant of these improper metabolic values. The Genius has become miss-programmed; it now thinks it is in a "healthy" state of health. As in hypoglycemia, when the Genius has become lazy in regulating those cells of the pancreas responsible for insulin production, we have a chronic condition which we choose to name "diabetes".

At this degenerative stage rest assured that many other cells operate poorly and other symptoms manifest themselves at the organ and metabolic level; you now have poor Krebs/ATP cycle and cellular exhaustion, mal-assimilation, mal-absorption and poor detoxification and elimination, deficient protein synthesis, sluggish osmosis of water (dehydration), deficient oxygenation (hypoxia). There is chronic acidity and resulting acidosis; not only do you have incorrect pH levels, but because of inefficient flushing of cellular debris, you have accumulated acid ashes inside and between the cells. These conditions have led to infestations of bacteria and parasites (fungus, yeast and Candida), to "bad" fats (high cholesterol) and to lack of viscosity. Frequently there is crystallization of fats and other unassimilated debris into plaque and arthritis. Your food / nutrients assimilation and elimination is deficient; you have lost your healing energy, your healing force, and it's now a vicious cycle.

HOW BAC AWAKENS THE GENIUS WITHIN?

As per Hippocrates's advice: "Let thy food be thy medicine", all good foods have the potential to nourish and heal. For this healing to be a reality, the nutrients in the food we eat must be assimilated and absorbed within the cell wall in a sufficient and required quantity. With wrong food choice, aging, and other metabolic deficiencies, this becomes quite difficult to achieve and cellular disease takes over. Due to its extraordinary nutrients content and their bioavailability, BAC's nourishment potential is hundreds of times higher than ordinary foods and other sources of nutrients. BAC's combined nutritional values and high utilization properties deliver the culmination in cellular nutrition.

PROPERTIES AND CHARACTERISTICS OF BAC

Whole food. In natural and holistic nutrition it is certain that whole foods are the way nature meant for us to nourish ourselves and that quality, not quantity, counts. For example, a minuscule amount of Vitamin C as it occurs in the whole orange or green pepper is tremendously more nutritionally functional than a mega dose of isolated ascorbic acid.

Organic. The "Bio" in Bio-Algae Concentrates means that it is of a living organism, that it is not isolated or separated or synthetic or chemical. It is grown without the use of synthetic fertilizers, pesticides, and without antibiotics, growth hormones or other dangerous additives.

Micro food. This is a key characteristic of BAC that explains why such nutritional power can reside in such a small quantity. BAC contains microalgae that hold extraordinary nutritional value for their size. The microalgae in BAC are invisible to the naked eye while they deliver more nutrients than any visible food particle. Furthermore, they contain no extraneous material like fiber, fat, bulk, and water. That makes BAC extremely digestible, non toxic, and with minimal assimilation and elimination burden for the body. BAC is pure energy.

Complete. Most foods, like an apple, are whole within themselves. But an apple does not contain many of the required nutrients that we need to sustain life. BAC is not only whole, but it is also the most complete food on earth containing amounts of all daily required nutrients and thousands more. There are over 5,000 known nutrients in BAC including Vitamins A, B, C, D, E, and K, all known minerals and trace elements, all known amino acids, a full protein makeup, chlorophyll, an array of mixed carotenoid antioxidants, and thousands of enzymes.

Balance. There are four microalgae in BAC. Each is a whole food and is naturally balanced within itself as most food is. However, anytime you mix different foods together you must be concerned with the chemical interactions as per the science of food combination. For example, eating watermelon over a steak is a nutritional disaster that will cause digestion problems. It took 9 years of intensive research to formulate the optimum balance found in BAC, patiently selecting the most compatible algae amongst the thousands investigated.

Bioavailability. BAC has an exceptionally high overall utilization ratio with no resulting toxicity. For example, its human active proteins have a 98-99% net utilization ratio while its calcium has a net utilization ratio over 95%. Several of its nutrients, like beta carotene, alpha carotene, and astaxanthin, are proven to penetrate the blood brain barrier. This sort of bioavailability and net utilization is possible because of the mentioned previous characteristics – whole food, organic, complete, micro food, and balance.

Synergy. At the molecular level, synergy is real. Synergy is what makes a violinist a virtuoso and a string orchestra the Boston Philharmonic. Once the 5,000 nutrients in BAC are subjected to digestive enzymic breakdown, they further explode into 50,000 sub nutrients and millions of sub molecules synthesized during digestion as enzymes, proteins, and other molecules that are generated at the mouth as amylase, at the pancreas as protease, disassembled and re-organized further by the liver and assimilated into the bloodstream and distributed within seconds by the flow of blood across the entire body to nourish trillions of cells.

WHAT ARE THE BENEFITS OF CONSUMING BAC?

We are energy beings. We live off the energy that we derive from the foods we eat. When the cells of the body receive the nutrients and the resulting energy that they need, they, like a virtuoso, will perform their multitude of cellular metabolic activities – growth, repair, cleansing, regeneration, and much more. When each cell of the organ performs its job well, then the organ will have a fighting chance to perform its metabolic activities, such as blood sugar regulation by the pancreas. But as per the discussion above, let's not forget that cellular activities and organ metabolic functions are controlled by the endocrine system which itself is overseen by the Genius.

The nutrients in BAC efficiently nourish the cells of the body, including those cells of the brain that make up the "Genius". Several phytonutrients and pigments found in BAC, like beta carotene, alpha carotene, lutein, lycopene, and astaxanthin, have been proven in several human clinical trials to easily cross the blood brain barrier, the blood retinal barrier, the cerebellum wall, etc.

When the Genius within is awakened, like any good commander, its first mission will be to restore the balance within his team, the endocrine glands, the guardians of health. When the endocrine glands are tasked by the Genius they have

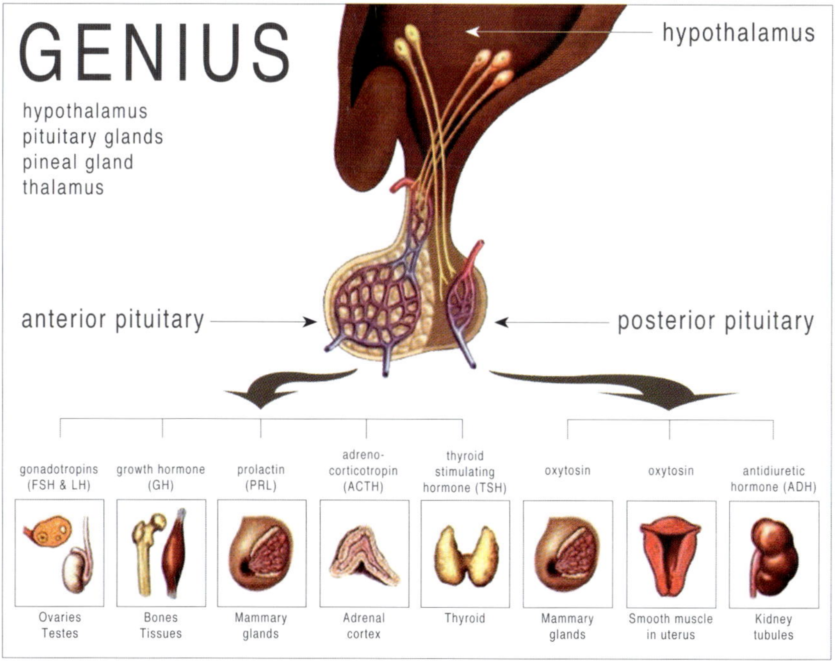

no choice but to obey the hormonal commands. These glands are in most part responsible for triggering the metabolic activity of the various organs and systems, such as blood insulin level, pH level, cardiac function, mineral activities, and myriads more. When we "Awaken the genius within", we improve the functions of our regulating organs and we replace the symptoms of disease with those of good health.

- Endocrine homeostasis
- Increased energy and energetic coherence
- Improved memory and neurologic function
- Improved cellular repair, including that of RNA and DNA
- Prevention of tumorigenesis
- Healthier cardiovascular system
- Balanced blood sugar and enhanced cellular glucose uptake
- Enhanced libido and fertility
- Reduced buildup of heavy and toxic metals
- Tangible feeling of wellness and renewal
- Increased immunity and protection from free radicals and diseases
- Increased assimilation, absorption, and elimination of consumed foods

THE MANY USES OF BAC

As discussed in this booklet, BAC is optimum nutrition and as such, is involved in many important body functions. It is almost unbelievable that a safe, natural substance, can be that effective for so many different types of conditions. Even I as the author was skeptical about BAC in the beginning. However, a thorough review of the scientific evidence, meeting with so many people, their health success stories, combined with an understanding of how BAC works in the body, makes it far easier to accept that BAC provides so many benefits.

For example, it becomes easy to comprehend why BAC is so safe when you know that algae have been created by Mother Nature billions of years ago and have always remained the "first" food. It's the food of plankton, small fish, and salmon. Microalgae are also known as "the bottom of the food chain" because they offer the most nutrients with the least toxicity per gram.

When fed the right raw materials, the human body has internal controls and mechanisms to keep it healthy and protected against damaging free radicals. BAC is one of those unsurpassed raw materials that allows witnessing this self-healing miracle in action.

Because of its involvement with most vital biochemical processes that affect human health, it is easy to understand why BAC can benefit a far wider range of conditions in addition to cancer. Over the years, Professor Kiriac has applied BAC successfully to treat many of our modern diseases and has shown the tremendous nutraceutical and therapeutic power of BAC in alleviating most degenerative diseases.

BAC now helps thousands of people in Europe, Canada and the USA, and provides health benefits for heart disease, cancer, diabetes, arthritis, fibromyalgia, liver disorders, osteoarthritis, glaucoma, endocrine gland disorders, depression, allergies, arthritis, nervous system and immune system disorders, anti-aging, sports and fitness, and many others.

NUTRITIONAL RECOMMENDATIONS

Doctor Kiriac recommends a comprehensive approach when dealing with illness, prevention, and treatment. BAC is not a panacea; you must also make efforts to improve all aspects of your life, including the physical and spiritual aspects. The most successful illness prevention and treatment program addresses diet, lifestyle factors like smoking, alcohol intake, stress, relationships, exercise and physical activity, and an awareness of the mind-body connection. In this context, BAC can make a profound difference. Nutrition-wise, Dr. Kiriac's recommendations for a healing rather than a demanding diet consist of:

- Never indulging in over-eating
- Choosing to eat mostly organic foods
- Eating whole and fresh foods (unprocessed)
- Eating mostly plants (varied greens, vegetables, and fruit) and some whole grains, beans, fish, eggs, lean meats, etc.
- Eating at least 50% raw or lightly cooked foods
- Not destroying the nutrients in your foods by overcooking
- Drinking at least 10 glasses of pure water everyday for basic hydration
- Making a concerted effort to eliminate all "junk" foods from your diet
- Exercising moderately everyday
- Think positively

Sound nutrition is not simple; it is both an art and a science. We must protect ourselves, immunize ourselves, and increase our basic protection with foods that are rich in enzymes, phytonutrients, essential fatty acids, vitamins, minerals, trace elements as only found in nature. Examples of these foods include: bee products such as bee propolis; fruit such as papaya and acerola; mushrooms like shiitake, reishi and maitake; grains, such as whole grain products, oat, lentils, mung beans, and basmati rice; sea vegetables like dulse, wakame, and hijiki; grasses, such as kamut and alfalfa; nutritional yeast; aloe vera; vinegars; alkalinizing fruit such as lemon, yellow grapefruit, and avocado; and many more.

But even with the best of nutrition and exercise, we remain under attack from several pollutants and other cancer-causing and bio-hazardous agents in our food, water, and air. We must further boost and protect ourselves and immunize ourselves with super micro-nutrients such as BAC, for this super natural protection. When making nutrition and supplementation choices, always seek advice from a professional and make certain to understand the recommendations in this booklet.

INTERNATIONAL RECOGNITION

In December 2001, as the highest educational honor of his life and career, Dr. Kiriac was nominated Professor of Education and Human Rights to Health by the International Association of Educators for International Peace and the International Consultative Organization. From that day forth, he holds the title of Professor or Professor Doctor Kiriac, to also honor his Doctorate. With this recognition, Professor Kiriac is entitled to teach at any French language university in Europe.

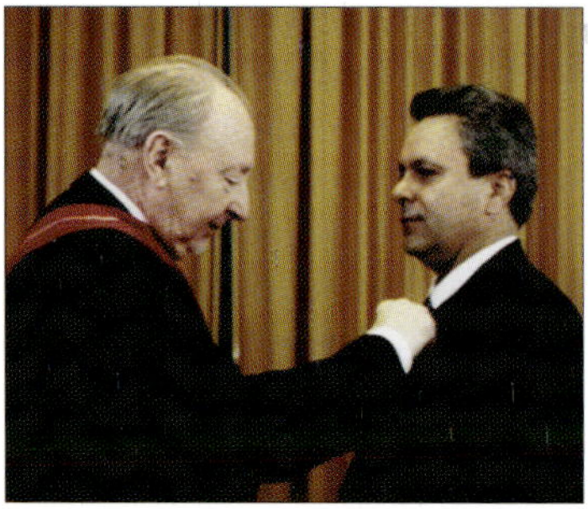

52ND EUREKA INTERNATIONAL INVENTION AWARD
Awards continue to abound for BAC and Dr. Kiriac

In November 2002, representing Canada, Dr. Kiriac was awarded honors at the 52nd Eureka International Invention conference held in Brussels, Belgium. BAC received the highest honors – the Commission's Cross and Golden Globe Award – BAC was hailed as the best Nutraceutical product in the world! Over 900 inventions from all over the world were presented at this annual show. As the rest of the world continues to recognize his work, Professor Kiriac is dedicated to work so that the miracle of BAC will assist the world towards better health and wellness.

Professor Kiriac continues to work closely with health practitioners and directly with patients as often as he can. He spends most of his time lecturing and training health practitioners that utilize BAC to help their clients in their practices. He continues his efforts to work closely with health sectors in Canada, providing training to doctors that are currently working with the product in their practice. BAC is sold in hundreds of vitamin and nutrition outlets and carried by hundreds of health practitioners.

SUMMARY OF AWARDS

- Nominated Moldova Person of the Year in 1987, Mr. Kiriac was nominated the person of the year in his country of Moldova for his resounding achievement and success at the most economically significant poultry center which provided considerable financial return for Moldova. A 150 minute's documentary film was made for the occasion and introduced on national television by Mr. Ciubuk, then Prime Minister of Moldova, and by the Minister of Finance.
- Gold Medal – New Technology for Algae Production – Iasi, Romania. This innovation was applied in the largest poultry farms of Moldova and was recognized at the International Exhibition for Research in Industrial Invention, 1994.
- Silver Medal – Element of Protein Synthesis – Pittsburgh USA. This innovation was well received and recognized during the Show Management Index sm IX., 1995.
- Gold Medal & Special Award – Earth Ecology – (Brussels, Belgium 1995) Industrial Use of Poultry Waste (Droppings). Invention honored and recognized during the International Eureka Show, granted by deheer Lue Van Den Bossch. The goal of this innovation was the elaboration of a new technology, which uses transformed poultry droppings at an industrial level.
- Nominated Professor (Education and Human Rights to Health) by the International Association of Educators for International Peace (AEIPM), and the International Consultative Organization (UNESCO, UNICEF, ECOSOC/ONU).
- Awarded Honorary Diploma in recognition of his international activities, in the social, humanitarian, cultural, scientific, health, education, and philanthropic domains. Award given by the International Association of Educators for International Peace (AEIPM), and the International Consultative Organization (UNESCO, UNICEF, ECOSOC/ONU).
- Nominated Doctor in Philosophy by the International Political and Cultural Sciences Academy – Brussels, Belgium, 2001.
- Gold Medal – Prof. Kiriac received for his efforts supporting the ills of Chernobyl with BAC, 2001.
- Gold Medal – Invention BAC for Animals – International Eureka 2002 – Brussels, Belgium
- Gold Medal Jury's Mention – Invention BAC – International Eureka 2001 – Brussels, Belgium
- Nominated Academician of Merits with Scientific Mention and Jury's special mention in recognition of his activities by the International Scientific Academy Life Universe Nature (A.S.I.V.U.N.) – Toulouse, France.
- Great Minds of the 21st Century – The Governing Board of Editors of the American Biographical Institute has selected Professor Kiriac as a Great Mind of the 21st Century due to his significant accomplishments within and mastery of Alternative Medicine. Documented in the premier edition of Great Minds of the 21st Century, reserved for Men and Women whose Accomplishments and Influences are the Results of Superior Conditioning of the Intellect.
- Cross of the Legion, Highest award from the Commission, 52nd Eureka 2002 Inventions and Technologies, Brussels, Belgium.